THE
BIG BENCH
PROGRAM!

How To Increase Your Bench Press By 50 Pounds In 30 Days!

By: Andrew Mitchell

www.BigBenchProgram.com

THE BIG BENCH PROGRAM
How To Increase Your Bench Press By 50 Pounds In 30 Days!

Address all inquiries to:
Andrew Mitchell
tel. (702) 701-4635
email: DestinedLegendz@gmail.com
www.DestinedLegendz.com

Cover Design: Marcus Richardson www.IonGrafix.com
DL DestinedLegendz Publishing
Las Vegas, NV 89117

ISBN-13: 978-1544626734
ISBN-10: 1544626738

Printed In The United States of America.

TABLES OF CONTENTS

ACKNOWLEDGMENTS

First and foremost, I thank God for everything because without God, I am nothing! Next, I dedicate this book to my Mom because she has always been my #1inspiration and guardian Angel. God rest her soul! I would also like to thank my fiancé, Ashley for being patient and understanding of me when I disappear into my office for hours to write! My big brother, Christopher, I thank you for helping me grow up, teaching me what you know, and for being my best coach and training partner ever! Arnold Schwarzenegger, thank you for inspiring me and helping me make my dreams of becoming a successful bodybuilder come true! And to ALL you passionate, hungry people out there who bust your butt, day in and day out, to be GREAT, I thank you for giving me a reason to write! BE BLESSED, and ALWAYS REMEMBER:

"IF IT WAS EASY, EVERYONE WOULD DO IT!"

THE

BIG BENCH

PROGRAM!

Inspired by two main intentions, I created this book. Since the most common question among regular gym buffs everywhere is, "What's your bench?" or "How much can you bench?" I felt it absolutely necessary to share my personalized strength building routine I created for myself, after years and years of trial and error and from studying all the greats in the sport! Even as a bodybuilder, 2-3x a year, I structured and dedicated my program to building strength! Sharing my journey of how I went from being a 96 lb. runt, feeling like the 'ugly-duckling' to becoming the nationally ranked competitive bodybuilder I became is very rewarding for me.

The second of my intentions became very clear to me after answering this sincere question I asked myself:

"What or how can I give back to the sport of bodybuilding?"

The, sometimes, harsh and brutally honest sport of bodybuilding is the lifestyle I chose to live and breathe for the past twenty-three years. This sport has taken so much from me, yet it has given me so much more in return. One thing I absolutely love about bodybuilding is no matter what kind of day I was having, or whatever was on my mind, *bodybuilding always remained the same!* It wore no masks. It told no lies. It was just me and the weights. The gym does not discriminate between sexes and races. One simple universal law applies:

You Get What You Give!

Just recently, I stood in the gym, in front of one of the mirrors that has reflected my image so many times before, yet, this time, I saw something different. I saw a man who has achieved a lot with his life, who no longer had aspirations to be THE BIGGEST or the strongest man, but a man - calm, powerful, and confident as ever who, now, wanted to give something back. I boldly confronted the intimidating image in the mirror, who fearlessly stared back directly into my eyes. After a dramatic pause, *and without answering*, he proceeds to ask me the exact same question I asked of him just moments before:

"What do I do, now?"

In a deep, meditative state of self-reflection, I stood frozen. Was I afraid to answer the question, or was I just not ready to? I believe we all want to leave our mark on the world and be remembered for something noble and virtuous, *something great!* And when we stand at the edge of our last step, we ask ourselves, "Did I leave my mark? Will I be remembered?"

That's exactly where I was on that day. Making the decision to retire from a career that I had been associated with from the time I was a teenager made me a little leery. I'd be lying if I said I was completely over bodybuilding. I'll always be in it, and it will always be in me. That being said, this is not "Good-bye… Just a 'See you later!"

When I first started working out, I was

barely able to BENCH PRESS the 45lb. bar for 10 reps. Willing to do whatever it took to change, I became obsessed, and completely consumed. Ten years later, I bench pressed 405lbs. 3x! This is one chapter of my beautiful story! Enjoy.

Introduction:

From the days of Eugen Sandow, to Charles Atlas, to Arnold, to the present-day greats of 'The World's Strongest Man' competitions, we, humans, have been driven to be big and strong! Normal is boring! Through the crowded halls of high schools and colleges to the weight rooms, and gyms world-wide, everyone wants to know the secrets of building a HUGE armor-plated chest and an incredible 'BENCH' to go with it!

What's more impressive than taking your shirt off to reveal a big, pumped up chest? Or, how intoxicating is it to gather around 'The Bench Press' with your closest iron brothas? One by one, you start stacking 45lb. iron plates onto the cold, steel bar, and as 3, then 4 plates go on each side, people start to stare! Adrenaline starts surging through your veins as you mount the bench. You grip the bar and plant yourself firmly underneath it. You hear the instrumental sounds of heavy metal music pounding in your ear drums. But nothing can drown out the sound of the warrior within you as your heartbeat echoes louder and louder…

"KILL THAT SHIT, MITCHELL!" I can still hear the order my buddy screams, just before punching me in the chest and smacking the side of my head, getting me insanely focused and prepared to lift 405lbs.

I break the small ammonia capsule I had been holding, take a big whiff from it, then, throw it to the ground. Shaking my head like a madman, I get in place, position my hands, and plant my feet. I lock in my arch and receive the lift-off. As my training partner let go of the bending piece of metal, it felt like the weight of the world was resting in my hands.

I embrace this rare opportunity because I am fully aware that: "I am one of the lucky ones…" My eyes were like lasers, insanely focused and able to easily penetrate through diamonds. In a visual image I had seen over and over countless times,

I lower the bar in a controlled manner, coiling my body like a spring, or better yet, a cobra about to attack! As it touches my vein-popping chest, I EXPLODE that bar upward, as though I'm being thrust through a canon! The bar moves effortlessly like a piston. I hear the chanting and cheering of the guys nearby, watching this incredible feat! Inspired by their admiration, I lower and press it up 2 more times!!! 405lbs for 3 REPS!!!

"WHEWWWWWW!"

I jump to my feet and slam my hands together like 2 brass cymbals colliding in a BIG CRESCENDO of an orchestra, and clouds of chalk explode into the air like an atomic bomb! "HELLYEAAA!" I scream as my boy wraps his giant arms around me and congratulates me on my new P.R. - PERSONAL RECORD.

That day was in 2005. I was just 24 years old, and I felt like He-Man. Later that year, as a Light-Heavyweight, weighing 197lbs, I'd go onto take 2nd place at 'The Ohio State Bodybuilding Championships', qualifying for my first ever National Bodybuilding Championships! The strength routine I'm about to share with you is the exact program I used to achieve my personal best ever bench press!

Mistakes People Make:

If you want to build a bigger bench that captures the attention of everyone in the gym, there are a few mistakes you need *NOT* to make. Too many people who aspire to build a beautiful body and drastically increase their strength make these mistakes that can halt your progress and potentially injure you!

1.) The #1 mistake people make is
   OVERTRAINING!

I understand the idea of, "If I train more often, I'll build my body and get stronger quicker!" That's true and false at the same time. It's true in the sense that you're going to achieve quicker results if you train 4 or 5 days a week, opposed to 2, "IF" you structure your program the correct way. What do I mean by that?

For example, I've seen guys set off on the quest for building a bigger bench press, and they have all the enthusiasm in the world, which is great and also necessary! However, the mistake they make is training chest or bench pressing *every single day*!   That's a quick way to get burned out and injured! As, I always say, "Even God rested 1 day!"

That's why it's incredibly IMPORTANT to properly design your workout programs. Always make sure you include auxiliary exercises that will help facilitate strong opposing muscle groups, as well as strengthening your stabilizer muscles, especially along your shoulder girdle. Follow the routine I've outlined here, and I promise you, your weight in the BENCH PRESS, (and ALL LIFTS) will *drastically* increase, in as little as 4 weeks!

2.) The #2 mistake people make is **NOT TRAINING LEGS!**

Heavy squats, 1,000lb leg presses, 25 rep sets of leg curls, leg extensions, step-ups, and 100 repetitions of walking lunges is not easy, so, most people avoid them altogether. We've all seen these guys in the gym. They always wear sweatpants or knee-high socks and baggy shorts to hide the fact that they have scrawny, little girl, *"chicken legs"!*

One, it's not attractive. Two, it's hard to respect a man (boy) who's afraid to get in the squat rack and squat til you puke! If you're going to be "A BOSS" in the gym and get your bench to an extreme level, capturing the attention of all the admirers, you have to build a respectable squat and deadlift, too! They don't have to be world record level, but they do *need* to be respectable!

Also, our legs make up at least half of our bodyweight, so if you serious about getting big and strong, you absolutely must train your legs! You will quickly see that as you build your legs and core strength, your bench will get even bigger! One reason is because squats and deadlifts release a natural spike and surge of growth hormone and testosterone, 2 of 3 main anabolic hormones in your body responsible for big muscles and incredible strength!

3.) The #3 mistake people make is **using bad form!!**

This makes me want to SCREAM!!! When you're bouncing the bar off your chest and lifting your ass off the bench like a caged gorilla trying to bang Pamela Anderson, you look like a dufus! And you're risking injury, as well. Not to mention, these are not real gainz!

Watch a legit powerlifting competition. These BEASTS, not only control the bar down, they even –pause- for a second before throwing it back up to their spotters! This is real strength and power! This is what you're after, and this is what I'm teaching!

Some suggestions I have here regarding proper form and safety, taught to me by a couple world record holders, are:

- Use chalk
- Use wrist straps
- Use elbow wraps
- Use a belt (optional)
- Use a spotter
- Proper Form: Plant feet firmly. Lock in "your grip". (Find what's most comfortable for you!) Create a big, strong arch, and lock it in!
- Tighten, "FLEX", your entire body
- Get a "lift-off"
- Control the bar down to a point on your chest. (Bar placement or the location of the

bar when it touches your chest may vary depending upon if you're training for strength or focusing on building muscle.) For strength or power, the bar position is usually a little lower on your chest. For overall development of your pec muscles, you can adjust the bar to a higher point (mid-chest) on your chest, targeting a slightly different area. When "maxing out", always use the same grip and bar position as you did previously!

- Once you touch the bar to your chest, EXPLODE! Explosively as possible, push that bar back up to the starting, or 'lock-out" position!

Nutrition:

We've all heard, "You are what you eat!" However, so few of us actually utilize this principle. If what we put in is what we get out, if we pollute our bodies with shitty food, we're going to look and feel shitty. If we feed ourselves healthy, healing, and energetic foods, we're going to be strong, healthy, and energetic! It's not rocket science! It's simple health 101.

Hopefully, we all have enough common sense to distinguish what's healthier for us. Here, let's practice. What provides more nutrition, an apple or French fries? What provides more high quality protein and less fat, 3 slices of greasy bacon or a grilled chicken breast? Which of these is a better source of fiber and complex carbohydrates, Fruit Loops or a bowl of old-fashioned oatmeal? See, you know more than you thought you did! Select smart food choices!

If you are totally clueless about what to eat, when and why, or if you just want professional guidance to get the best results possible, go to my website www.DestinedLegendz.com and purchase a customized meal plan. You'll be guided to fill out a questionnaire regarding your goals and lifestyle habits, and I will create the ideal nutrition program for you to maximize your results.

Here are a few basic nutrition tips:

- Eat at least 5-6 smaller food meals/protein shakes a day, opposed to 1-3 large meals.
- Cut out sweets and junk food.
- Drink at least 1 gallon of water a day.
- Eat at least 1 gram of protein per pound of bodyweight. If you're a hardgainer, eat 2 grams of protein per lb. of BW.
- If you want to gain weight, eat at least 2 grams of carbohydrates per pound of bodyweight. Hardgainers eat 3 grams per lb. of BW.
- Take a good multi-vitamin/mineral supplement, every day!
- Add 5-10 grams of creatine, glutamine, and BCAAs to your workout program

Proper Mindset:

If the food we eat is the fuel for our bodies, our thoughts are the gears and catalysts that create motion, not the body, alone. "Our bodies only do what the mind first tells it to do!" Let's look at it like this: Our bodies are high operating machines like a Ferrari. First, we have to take care of it, (food), with routine oil changes, brake inspections, etc, and give it the highest quality and octane of fuel available. So, we have this body that is primed and ready for the road, but if we don't have a driver for the car, (our mind), it just sits there and collects dust. We need a driver and a good driver at that!

So, we're committed to working out, but we've become lazy or lackadaisical, and we've hit a plateau. But you're ready to change! Your champion mindset is what you're going to use in the gym and out in the world every day to show the universe just how powerful you are!

For 10-15min, before every workout, hop on the treadmill and get the blood flowing through your body. Also, do some light calisthenics to 'warm-up" and continue loosening up your body. As well as to shake off any bad energy or stress you may have had from the day, use this time effectively to visualize your workout. See yourself performing at your highest level! Imagine yourself as SUPER-HUMAN, because you are! *Aren't you?*

> "Others tend to take you at your own self-evaluation!" –Norman Vincent Peale
> *And...*
> "As a man thinks in his heart, so is he!"
> –Proverbs 23:7

Set your goals for the workout. You know what you're there to achieve and why? *Do not let anything OR anyone distract you.* You're a lion! You're a fucking beast! You're not afraid of the storm. You are the storm! You are a destined legend, destined for greatness!

Always approach your workouts and your life like this, and you will amaze yourself at how powerful you truly are!

"Where emotion goes, energy flows!"
–Tony Robbins

From years of studying people, reading and attending personal growth seminars, and by analyzing myself, I have become confidently aware of the power we have within ourselves in determining our *success or failure*, in life! If you do not take charge of your thoughts, as you get physically stronger, your own mind will begin questioning you. When you start breaking your own P.R.'s, you must constantly feed yourself powerful thoughts and affirmations, or weak, self-defeating thoughts such as these will take over:

- Wow! This is a lot of weight!
- You can't lift this much weight!
- You're not strong enough!
- You're gonna fail!

Never entertain that negative voice!
Defeat it with powerful thoughts, beliefs, and actions!

- "I *can* bench press 200lbs, 300lbs, 400lbs, 500lbs!"
- "I am a champion!"
- "I deserve success!"

You can do it! You will do it! Just know that achieving anything in life begins with believing in yourself and having the faith that you can do anything!

The Program:

The Percentages are only for The BENCH PRESS

Monday: **HEAVY DAY**
(80-90% of your 1RM – Rep Max)
Chest/Arms Emphasis:

Bench Press – 5x5   Do 1 warm-up set of 20 reps
with about 35% of your heaviest work set. (Round
weights to the nearest 5lb increment.) Perform
another warm-up set of 15 reps with about 50% of
your heaviest work set. Do a third warm-up set
with about 75% of your heaviest work set. Then,
complete 5 sets of 5 reps with 80-90% of your
1RM.

Incline DB Press – 4x20, 15, 12, 8-10

(Superset):
Leg Press – 4x12-15
Walking Lunges – 4x20 steps (10 steps down/10
steps back)

(Superset):
Standing DB Biceps Curls – 4x20
Skull Crusher/Close-grip Bench Combo – 4x15, 10, 8,8

Notes:

Tuesday: CARDIO DAY
Calves/Abs:

Do 20-30min of light to moderate cardio on treadmill.
(Incline Intervals or jogging)
Calves superset:
Standing calf raises and Seated calf raises – 3x15-20
Abs giant set:
Sit-ups and kick-ups 3x20 and Planks – 3x60 sec

STRETCH!

Notes:

Wednesday: **LIGHT DAY**
(60-70% of 1RM)
Legs Emphasis:

Bench Press – 5x5 (use same protocol and percentages as Monday. Just be sure the 35/50/75% is your 60-70% of your 1RM.)

Squats – 5x20, 15, 12, 10, 8

(Superset):
Dips and Push-ups – 3xMAX REPS

(Superset):
Lying leg curls and Leg extensions – 3x15-20

Notes:

Thursday: CARDIO DAY

Calves/Abs:

Do 20-30min of light to moderate cardio on treadmill.

(Incline Intervals or jogging)

Calves superset:

Standing calf raises and Seated calf raises 3x15-20

Abs giant set:

Sit-ups and kick-ups 3x20 and Planks – 3x60 sec

STRETCH!

Notes:

Friday: **MEDIUM DAY**
(70-80% of 1RM)
Back and Shoulders Emphasis:

Bench Press – 5x5

Deadlifts - 5x5

(Superset):
Pull-Ups – 4xMax Reps/Push-Ups – 4x25

(Superset):
Bent-over Rows/Military Presses – 4x8-12

(Superset):
DB Lateral raises/DB Shrugs – 4x20/15/12/10

Notes:

Overview:

This is an old-school approach to strength training. There are no short-cuts, miracle drugs, or special formulas that will take the place of hard work, discipline, and commitment! Nowadays, people want results overnight without doing the work. If it was easy, everyone would be rich, powerful, and sexy. And, if so, then, these qualities would not be so honorable, and the pay-off and reward of achieving them would not be so great!

Success is a choice! So is failure. If you want something bad enough, you have to sacrifice time, money, and energy! How valuable are your dreams to you? Make a decision right now to always go all out, and you will be successful!

Best Wishes,
Drew Mitchell
CEO DestinedLegendz LLC